Vegetarian Bodybuilding Nutrition;
How to Crack the Muscle-Building Success Code with Vegetarian Bodybuilding Nutrition, 21 Muscle Building Recipes
By
Greg Fordham

All Rights Reserved. No part of this publication may be reproduced in any form or by any means, including scanning, photocopying, or otherwise without prior written permission of the copyright holder. Copyright © 2015

Table of Contents

1. Can you Build Muscle with a Vegetarian Diet?
2. Breakfast - Mega Eggs and Quinoa
3. Breakfast - Cinnamon Quinoa
4. Breakfast - Grab-N-Go Protein Hit
5. Breakfast - Protein-Packed Oatmeal
6. Breakfast - Muscle Building Pancake
7. Lunch - The Epic Tortilla
8. Lunch - Quinoa Carb Salad
9. Lunch - Mushroom and Quinoa Stack
10. Lunch - Pasta with Peppers
11. Lunch - Fat-free Stuffed Pasta Shells
12. Dinner - Quorn Mince Lasagne
13. Dinner - Ricotta Cheese Lasagne
14. Dinner - Tofu Chilli and Quinoa
15. Dinner - Macaroni Cheese
16. Dinner - Hot Tofu and Rice
17. Snack - Mexican Black Beans and Avocado
18. Snack - Raisin Oatmeal Cookie
19. Snack - Fast Yogurt and Apricot
20. Snack - Protein Banana Smoothie
21. Snack - Guacamole Hummus
22. Snack - Sweet Cinnamon Quinoa Punch
23. Snack - Protein Apple and Celery Smoothie
24. The Number One Mistake to Avoid!

1. Can you Build Muscle with a Vegetarian Diet?

Building muscle is a combination of hard training and nutrition. Put like that it sounds very simple. To go one step further with nutrition - you must consume more calories than you are burning in a day - everyday. Otherwise there is no fuel to build muscle and you will never ever grow. Bodybuilding nutrition whether you want an extra two inches on your arms to add 25lbs of muscle is all about the food you ingest. Most people know how to workout. But it's nutrition we fall down on.

So what calories should we be consuming? A mix of protein, carbs and fats. The ratios vary from expert to expert and, but i go for a 40% Protein, 40% Carbs and 20% Fats. These figures can vary body to body. It's up to you to try things out and see how your body reacts. Okay simple, but what if you don't want to eat red meat and chicken? You actually care about the animals and environment? How do you consume enough high quality protein to GROW muscles?

Well it's not as hard as it sounds!

Today we have we as vegetarians actually have a huge array of protein-packed alternatives to meat that are not only jammed with nutrients for building muscle but taste GREAT! Some of these are commonly known, others are not so well known.

Not only will you find 21 recipes from breakfast to dinner, but also protein shakes, snacks and I encourage you to swap out ingredients to get creative.

I'm also forever adding a little punch to post-workout meals:
- Adding more whole or egg whites
- A table spoon of natural Peanut Butter.
- Three table spoons of Cottage Cheese
- Handful of Cashew Nuts

Obviously eggs and diary are a great source of protein (if you eat them). But here is a fantastic list of other high-protein Vegetarian foods to utilize in your meals that I include in my recipes.

MYCOPROTEIN (QUORN)
Protein: 13 grams per 1/2 cup serving

SOY
Protein: 10 grams per 1/2 cup serving (firm tofu); 15 grams per 1/2 cup serving (tempeh); 15 grams per 1/2 cup serving (natto)

QUINOA
Protein: 8 grams per 1 cup serving, cooked

BUCKWHEAT
Protein: 6 grams per 1 cup serving, cooked

HEMPSEED
Protein: 10 grams per 2 tablespoon serving

CHIA
Protein: 4 grams per 2 tablespoon serving

EZEKIEL BREAD
Protein: 8 grams per 2 slice serving

SEITAN
Protein: 21 grams per 1/3 cup serving

SPIRULINA WITH GRAINS OR NUTS
Protein: 4 grams per 1 tablespoon

HUMMUS AND PITA
Protein: 7 grams per 1 whole-wheat pita and 2 tablespoons of hummus

PEANUT BUTTER SANDWICH
Protein: 15 grams per 2-slice sandwich with 2 tablespoons of peanut butter

Without further ado let's get to the receipts. Don't forget to read the last Chapter where i reveal the number one mistake people make when building muscle on a vegetarian diet!

2. Breakfast - Mega Eggs and Quinoa

This is a hard-hitting breakfast - packed with a whopping 44grams of protein and a healthy dose of carbs if you have the side dish - ideal before or after a workout or to see you through to Lunch.

INGREDIENTS

- 225g - firm Tofu (chopped or crumbled)
- 3 - Egg Whites
- 1 - Whole Egg
- 2 - cups Spinach
- 1/2 - cup sliced Mushrooms
- 1/2 - cup Cherry Tomatoes
- Olive Oil, fresh Garlic, Soy Sauce, Lemon Juice and Salt and Pepper.

DIRECTIONS

Whisk the egg and egg whites together in a jug.
Add tomatoes, mushrooms, and 1 clove of garlic (crushed or chopped) into warmed frying pan and cook until the mushrooms have softened, turning slightly golden brown.
Add egg mixture to frying pan with tomatoes and mushrooms, stirring occasionally.

Tip - I like to sieve the egg mix as I pour it into the frying pan or saucepan. This removes all the gooey bits haha - try it and see if you approve.

As the scrambled eggs begin to set - Turn the heat to low and add the tofu, a splash of soy sauce, splash of lemon, and your salt and pepper to taste.
Cook letting some of the liquid cook off and the tofu to warm up.

Turn off the heat and mix in the spinach.

3. Breakfast - Cinnamon Quinoa

INGREDIENTS

- 1/4 cup cooked Quinoa
- 1 palm-full of Walnuts or Pecans
- 1 palm-full of Blackberries or Blueberries
- Sprinkle of Cinnamon
- Sweeten with Stevia (zero-calorie natural sweetener) or use agave nectar or some soft Honey.

DIRECTIONS

Cook your Quinoa in a saucepan of boiling for water for 15 minutes (you can add a splash of soy milk, almond milk, or hemp milk if you want it to be moister).
Drain the water from the Quinoa and put into a separate large bowl.
Add the walnuts, blackberries, cinnamon and Stevia and mix it all together with a spoon.

NUTRITION

Serving Size (including Quinoa on the side)
Amount per serving
- Calories 418
- Total Fat 26g
- Total Carbs 29g
- Protein 44g

4. Breakfast - Grab-N-Go Protein Hit

This is a time-efficient Breakfast - prepare the night before - grab and go in the morning with a heavy duty 22 grams of protein.

INGREDIENTS

- 1/4 - cup Rolled Oats
- 1/2 - cup Almond Milk
- 1/2 - scoop Chocolate Protein Powder
- 1 - Large Spoon of Natural Yogurt
- 1 - Banana
- 1 - tbsp Chia Seeds
- 1/2 - tbsp Cinnamon

DIRECTIONS

Mix all ingredients together in a large bowl - slice banana on top and add more Protein powder and Yogurt if additional protein is needed.
Once finished place in plastic container in fridge overnight.
Grab and go in the morning for a fast start to the day.

The easy thing with this is you can take away the oats if you just want a protein hit and this becomes a mid-morning snack. Add more honey to it to spike insulin levels and it becomes the perfect post workout hit.

NUTRITION

Recipe serves 1
Amount per serving
- Calories 306
- Total Fat 15.6 g
- Total Carb 32.1 g
- Protein 22.7 g

5. Breakfast - Protein-Packed Oatmeal

The classic porridge/oatmeal breakfast - easy to prepare - excellent slow carbs 29 grams - big on 23 grams of protein with added powder.

INGREDIENTS

- 1/4 - cup Rolled Oats
- 1/4 - cup berries, choose your preference (I used Blueberries)
- 1/2 - cup water - or Oat Milk, Soya Milk, Coconut Milk - you're choice!
- 1/2 - scoop Protein Powder - choose your preference
- 1 - tbsp all-natural Peanut Butter

DIRECTIONS

Place the berries in a microwave-safe bowl and microwave for 30 seconds.
Remove and smash the berries with a fork.
Add oats, water, and protein powder.
Microwave the mixture for 1.30 minutes - then stir - microwave for another 1 minute.

Stir and top with peanut butter if you want even more protein. Or add more protein powder, but it can become a little thick with too much. Also I've found i have to add more water/milk after the first microwave.

In a Saucepan
This does taste better - Add oats and water/milk and protein powder to a saucepan - stir and heat up until it starts to boil. Then leave it for 5 minutes stirring occasionally. Then reheat and serve.

NUTRITION

Recipe serves 1
Amount per serving
- Calories 317
- Total Fat 12.7 g
- Total Carb 29.4 g
- Protein 23.6 g

6. Breakfast - Muscle Building Pancake

A little more time is required - but very tasty - and at 33 grams of protein and 30 grams of superb carbs it's a great start to the day.

INGREDIENTS

- 6 - Egg Whites
- 1/2 - cup Oats
- 1 - scoop Protein Powder (Any Flavour)
- 1/2 - cup of flour
- 2 - tbsp Sugar-free Pancake syrup

DIRECTIONS

Mix the egg whites, oats, flour and Protein Powder in a jug. Heat a non-stick pan over medium-high heat and coat with 0 cal non-stick spray.
Pour 1/4 cup of the pancake batter into the pan and let cook until bubbles begin to appear. Pour more mixture. Flip and cook on the other sides until firm.
Serve with the syrup.

If you're feeling creative why not add some blue berries to the mix - they taste great!

NUTRITION

Serving Size: 2
Amount per serving
- Calories 292
- Total Fat 5g
- Total Carbs 30g
- Protein 33g

7. Lunch - The Epic Tortilla

Not for the faint hearted! Will need preparing before work if not at home - an epic lunch of 32 grams of protein.

INGREDIENTS

- 1 - 8 Inch Whole Tortilla
- 1 - Whole Egg
- 3 - Egg Whites
- 1 - Lettuce Leaf
- 2 - tbsp kidney Beans
- 1 - tbsp reduced-fat grated Cheese
- 1/4 - cup Salsa

DIRECTIONS

Lightly coat a medium non-stick frying pan with cooking spray and place over medium heat. Place tortilla in the frying pan and warm for 30 seconds, then flip and warm the other side for 30 seconds. Place the warmed tortilla on a small plate.
Whisk the egg and egg whites together. Pour into the frying pan and cook, stirring occasionally, until set.
Place the lettuce leaf on the tortilla and spread the kidney beans over the lettuce leaf. Top the beans with the cooked eggs, add grated cheddar cheese, and 2 tablespoons of salsa.
Roll it up and top with remaining salsa.

Tip - Why not cut it up into sections and use it as a super snack before and after the gym.

NUTRITION

Serving Size: 1 serving
Amount per serving
- Calories 313
- Total Fat 10g
- Total Carbs 30g
- Protein 32g

8. Lunch - Quinoa Carb Salad

A small and quick lunch jammed full of goodness.

INGREDIENTS

- 1 - cup Quinoa
- 1 - cup Soy Beans
- 1 - Red Bell Pepper
- 1/4 - cup chopped Coriander
- 1 - Lime
- 1 - tbsp Olive Oil
- 1/2 - tbsp each of Garlic Powder, Onion Powder, Cumin, and Paprika
- Salt and Pepper, to taste

Optional Add-ins
- 1/2 - cup cooked Black Beans
- 1/2 - chopped Red Onion
- 1 - chopped Tomato
- 1/2 - chopped Cucumber
- 1/4 - cup Hummus
- A dollop of Peanut Butter to increase healthy fats and protein

DIRECTIONS

Cook Quinoa for about 5 mins - depending how soft you like it could be up to 15minutes. Reduce to a simmer and cover. Remember Quinoa soaks up a lot of water so you may have to keep topping it up.
In a separate small saucepan, boil Soy Beans in water until fully cooked (check packaging) If you cook the beans the night before this makes it very quick

Once Quinoa and Soy beans are fully cooked, add all ingredients in a large bowl and mix until all flavors are combined.

NUTRITION

Serving Size Per serving, recipe makes 4 servings
Amount per serving
- Calories 141
- Total Fat 6g
- Total Carbs 16g
- Protein 12g

9. Lunch - Mushroom and Quinoa Stack

A Quorn and Quinoa punch that delivers a solid 18 grams of Vegetable Protein.

INGREDIENTS

- 2 - large Mushroom Portabella Caps rinsed clean and dried
- 1 - cup cooked Quinoa
- 1/2 - cup crumbled Tempeh OR Quorn Pieces
- 1/2 - Onion, diced
- 1 - cup Spinach
- 1 - Tomato, sliced
- 2 - tbsp grated Cheese OR fat-free Mozzarella
- 1 - tbsp Olive Oil
- 1/2 - tbsp each of Paprika, Cumin, Garlic Powder, and Onion Powder

Add Sea Salt and Black Pepper.

DIRECTIONS

Pre heat oven at 180C
Heat olive oil in a large pan over medium heat.
Add onion and Tempeh/Quorn to pan and sauté for 2-3 minutes, or until onion begins to soften.
Add Quinoa, spices, salt and pepper and sauté a few more minutes.
On a baking sheet, place Portobello mushrooms brushed lightly with olive oil.
Stack mushroom caps with spinach, Quinoa mixture, sliced tomatoes, and grated cheese.
Cook for 5 minutes in pre heated oven.

Tip - I often make double the portion and have this the next day.

NUTRITION

Serving Size: 2
Amount per serving
- Calories 324
- Total Fat 14g
- Total Carbs 34g
- Protein 18.25g

10. Lunch - Pasta with Peppers

Delicious 43 gram carb meal - perfect for a pre-workout energy boost.

INGREDIENTS

- 1 - cup fresh sliced Mushrooms
- 3 - chopped Onions
- 1 - large Green Pepper - cut into strips
- 3 - cups uncooked Rigatoni - *go for gluten free*
- 1 - jar (24 oz.) chunky spaghetti sauce
- 1 - cup Shredded Italian Mozzarella-Parmesan Cheese Blend

DIRECTIONS

Heat oven to 190C. Sauté onions, peppers, and mushrooms for 5 minutes, or until cooked through. Meanwhile, cook pasta as directed on package. So really you want it soft, but not too soft!
Drain pasta and add pepper & mushroom mixture to baking dish with spaghetti sauce; stir. Bake 15 to 20 minutes until heated through. Top with cheese; bake 2 to 3 minutes or until melted.

NUTRITION

Servings 6
Amount Per Serving
- Calories: 282.2
- Total Fat: 7.3 g
- Total Carbs: 43 g
- Protein: 11.9 g

11. Lunch - Fat-free Stuffed Pasta Shells

The perfect lunch or snacks on the go - 4 shells = 23 grams of protein.

INGREDIENTS

- 12 - Jumbo Shell Pastas
- 110g - fat-free Cream Cheese
- 170g - fat-free Cottage Cheese
- 1 - cup fat-free shredded Mozzarella
- 1 - cup chopped Mushrooms
- 2 - cups Marinara sauce
- 3 - tsp granulated Garlic
- 1/2 - tbsp dried Oregano
- 1/2 - tbsp dried Parsley
- 1 - tsp dried Rosemary

DIRECTIONS

Pre heat oven to 180C.
Boil jumbo pasta shells in a saucepan until they are nearly done -- al dente.
Drain and rinse under cold water. Set aside.
Mix all the cream cheese, cottage cheese, mozzarella cheese, mushrooms and spices in a large bowl.
With a spoon - pack pasta shells with cheese mixture.
Place each stuffed pasta shell into an oven-safe high sided container.
Pour marinara evenly over stuffed shells.
Cover with foil and place into oven for about 20 minutes.

NUTRITION

Servings: 4
Amount Per Serving
- Calories: 281.0
- Total Fat: 1.7 g
- Total Carbs: 38.6 g
- Protein: 27.4 g

12. Dinner - Quorn Mince Lasagne

Who can resist a hearty helping of Quorn Lasagne at 19grams of protein?

INGREDIENTS

- 3 - Cups Quorn Mince
- 1 - Medium Onion
- 1 - tbsp Garlic powder
- 1 - tin Canned Tomatoes
- 1 - cup of Water
- 8 - Lasagne sheets
- 1 - tbsp Parsley
- 1 - tbsp Basil
- 1 - tbsp ground Oregano
- 1 - cup Fat free Cottage Cheese
- 0.25 - cup reduced fat grated Parmesan cheese
- 1 - cup Spaghetti Sauce

DIRECTIONS

Pre heat oven at 180C.
In a frying pan cook the Quorn mince following packets instructions.
Add onion, garlic, tomatoes and spaghetti sauce, Stir in parsley, basil, and oregano.
In oven-proof dish layer in Lasagne sheets and mince mixture.
Spread Cottage cheese over top layer and sprinkle grated Parmesan cheese on top.
Cook in oven for 20 minutes.

NUTRITION

Servings: 4
Amount Per Serving
- Calories: 290.9
- Total Fat: 5.0 g
- Total Carbs: 43.9 g
- Protein: 19.5 g

13. Dinner - Ricotta Cheese Lasagne

A twist on the Lasagne with delicious Ricotta Cheese 40 grams of carbs and 20 grams of Protein.

INGREDIENTS

- 400g - of Ricotta Cheese
- 1 - Medium Onion
- 1 - tbsp Garlic powder
- 1 - tin Canned Tomatoes
- 1 - cup of Water
- 8 - Lasagne sheets
- 1 - tbsp Parsley
- 1 - tbsp Basil
- 1 - tbsp ground Oregano
- 0.25 - cup reduced fat grated Parmesan cheese
- 1 - cup Spaghetti Sauce

DIRECTIONS

Pre heat oven at 180C.
Mix all ingredients in a large bowl except Lasagne sheets.
In oven-proof dish layer in Lasagne sheets and above mixture.
Sprinkle grated Parmesan cheese on top.
Cook in oven for 20 minutes.

NUTRITION

Servings: 4
Amount Per Serving
- Calories: 290.9
- Total Fat: 7.0 g
- Total Carbs: 43.9 g
- Protein: 20.5 g

14. Dinner - Tofu Chilli and Quinoa

A two-serving beast at 27 grams of protein per serving.

INGREDIENTS

- 1 - cup Quinoa
- 1/4 - cup Brown sugar
- 1/4 -cup Soy sauce
- 1 - tsp Chili sauce
- 2 - tsp Sesame oil
- 2 - minced garlic cloves
- 1 - tsp grated fresh ginger
- Pinch of sea salt
- 340g - Tofu
- 1 - tsp olive oil

DIRECTIONS

Cook Quinoa as directed on the packet.
Mix brown sugar, soy sauce, chili sauce, sesame oil, garlic cloves, ginger and sea salt in a small bowl and set aside.
Pour olive oil into sauce pan and heat.
Fry Tofu in pan for about 10 minutes.
Pour sauce into pan and cook for 3-5 minutes. Sauce will thicken and the Tofu will absorb most of it.
Then add to Quinoa and mix thoroughly - allow to simmer for 5 minutes while stirring. Then it's ready to serve.

NUTRITION

Serves 2
Amount per serving
- Calories 329
- Total Fat 18 g
- Total Carbs 27 g
- Protein 27 g

15. Dinner - Macaroni Cheese

Simple pasta dish that tastes great and provides 45 grams of carbs and 19 grams of protein.

INGREDIENTS

- 220g - of pasta of choice
- 1/2 - cup milk (OR unflavored Coconut/Rice/Soya milk etc)
- 1/4 - cup unflavoured Pea Protein Powder
- 1/4 - cup grated Cheddar Cheese
- 1 - tbsp coconut flour
- 1 - tsp of Parmesan Cheese
- Garlic salt to taste
- Italian seasoning
- Dry Parsley OR Basil

DIRECTIONS

Cook the pasta of your choice until al dente.
Mix all of the milk, Pea Protein, Cheddar Cheese, Coconut Flour into a saucepan. Bring sauce to a simmer and continue to stir until all of the components are well combined and sauce thickens.
Drain water from pasta.
Add the sauce to your pasta, mix and simmer for 5 minutes stirring occasionally.

Serve and sprinkle with Parmesan cheese - absolutely perfect!

NUTRITION

Serving size: 4
Amount per serving
- Calories 271
- Total Fat 4 g
- Total Carbs 45 g
- Protein 19 g

16. Dinner - Hot Tofu and Rice

Spicy Tofu delivers an impressive 18 grams of protein.

INGREDIENTS

- 1 - package extra firm Tofu
- 2 - cups cooked Brown Rice
- 2 - tbsp Low-sodium Soy sauce
- 1 - tsp each of Ginger, Garlic Powder, and Onion Powder
- 1 - tsp Chili Paste
- 1 - bunch chopped Broccoli
- 1 - sliced Red Bell Pepper
- 1 - sliced Orange Bell Pepper

DIRECTIONS

Chop tofu into cubes.
Cook brown rice in a sauce pan of boiling water following packet instructions.
In a large sauce pan heat olive oil over medium heat.
Add broccoli and bell pepper and stir until lightly softened.
Heat another pan to medium heat and add Tofu.
Cook tofu for 5 minutes, stirring occasionally until all sides get cooked.
Serve brown rice and top with tofu, veggies, and green onions.

NUTRITION

Serving: 4
Amount per serving
- Calories 257
- Total Fat 8g
- Total Carbs 13g
- Protein 18g

17. Snack - Mexican Black Beans and Avocado

Perfect pre-workout snack giving you a hefty 40 grams of carbs.

INGREDIENTS

- 1/2 - cup cooked Brown Rice
- 1/3 - cup cooked Black Beans
- 2 - heaping spoonful's of Salsa
- 1/4 - sliced Avocado
- 2 - tbsp plain Fat-free Greek Yogurt

A hot sauce of your choosing or something like Sweet and Sour - just a dash.

DIRECTIONS

This is ideal if you have ingredients left over. Mix all ingredients in a large bowl - serve and enjoy.

NUTRITION

Serving Size 1
Amount per serving
- Calories 292
- Total Fat 9g
- Total Carbs 40g
- Protein 12g

18. Snack - Raisin Oatmeal Cookie

Did someone say cookies?

INGREDIENTS

- 1/2 - cup Rolled Oats
- 1 - Egg
- 11 g - of Unsweetened Applesauce
- 14 g - Raisins
- 1 - Tbsp Cinnamon
- 1 - Tbsp Stevia

DIRECTIONS

Preheat oven to 350.
Combine all the ingredients in a small bowl.
Pour into pre-sprayed Ramekins (small over-proof dish).
Place the Ramekins in the oven for 20 minutes, or until the oats are slightly toasted.

NUTRITION

Recipe serves 2
Amount per serving
- Calories 185
- Total Fat 4 g
- Total Carb 38 g
- Protein 6.6 g

19. Snack - Fast Yogurt and Apricot

A top-notch evening snack before bed to see you through the night with slow proteins and fats.

INGREDIENTS

- 220 g - of Greek Style Yogurt
- 1-2 - palm-fulls of raw or roasted Almonds (unsalted and unsweetened)
- 1 - palm-full of dried Apricot
- 1 - packet of Stevia (zero calorie sweetener) or a bit of agave or Honey

DIRECTIONS

Mix all the above ingredients in a large bowl - serve in a small bowl and eat up!

NUTRITION

Serving Size
Amount per serving
- Calories 428
- Total Fat 23g
- Total Carbs 31g
- Protein 23g

20. Snack - Protein Banana Smoothie

A stunning protein shake delivering 32 grams of protein.

INGREDIENTS

- 500ml - of Water
- 1 - Scoop of Rice Protein
- 1/2 - Scoop of Pea Protein
- 2 - Bananas
- 0.5 - cup skim milk (OR almond, soy, coconut, or cashew milk)
- 10 - Almonds
- 1 - Handful of Ice

DIRECTIONS

Add all the ingredients to a Blender and mix for 4 minutes. Pour into a shaker for on the go or a tall glass.

Tip - Don't neglect the ice - this really adds to the taste and density.

NUTRITION

Serving size: 1 shake
Amount per serving
- Calories 320
- Total Fat 8 g
- Total Carbs 32 g
- Protein 32 g

21. Snack - Guacamole Hummus

A great little dish giving you 22 grams of carbs - ideal with a protein shake.

INGREDIENTS

- 1 - can Chickpeas
- 1 - Avocado
- 1 - Jalapeano
- 1/4 - cup chopped cilantro
- Juice from 1 Lime

DIRECTIONS

Mix ingredients together in a large bowl until thoroughly mixed.
Then serve with vegetables, pita chips, or snack of your choice.

Combine with one of the smoothies for more of a protein hit.

NUTRITION

Serves 4
Amount per serving
- Calories 200
- Total Fat 9 g
- Total Carbs 22 g
- Protein 7.5g

22. Snack - Sweet Cinnamon Quinoa Punch

Walnuts and Quinoa mix to give you a 12grams of protein and 29 grams of carbs.

INGREDIENTS

- 1/4 - cup Quinoa
- 1 - palm-full of Walnuts or Pecans 7-10 individual nuts)
- 1 - palm-full of Blackberries or Blueberries
- Sprinkle of Cinnamon

Sweeten with Stevia (zero-calorie, natural sweetener) or use agave nectar or Honey

DIRECTIONS

Cook your Quinoa in a sauce pan as per instructions on packet. Drain once cooked.
Add the walnuts, blackberries, cinnamon and Stevia and mix it all together with a spoon. Serve hot!

NUTRITION

Serving Size 1
Amount per serving
- Calories 418
- Total Fat 26g
- Total Carbs 29g
- Protein 12g

23. Snack - Protein Apple and Celery Smoothie

The super shake - 32 grams of protein and 32 grams of carbs - no messing around here.

INGREDIENTS

- 500ml - of Water
- 1 - Scoop of Rice Protein
- 1/2 - Scoop of Pea Protein
- 1 - apple
- 2 - Sticks of Celery
- 0.5 - Cup of skim milk (OR almond, soy, coconut, or cashew milk)
- 10 - Almonds
- 1 - Handful of Ice

DIRECTIONS

Add all the ingredients to a Blender and mix for 4 minutes. Pour into Shaker for on the go or a tall glass.

Tip - As i said before always add the ice - really helps. You could also add a dollop of peanut butter instead of the almonds if you preferred.

NUTRITION

Serving size: 1 shake
Amount per serving
- Calories 320
- Total Fat 8 g
- Total Carbs 32 g
- Protein 32 g

24. The Number One Mistake to Avoid!

So what is the number one mistake I hear you cry? It's very simple - Preparation.

One of the biggest mistakes people make is not planning ahead and this is crucial to building muscle. Letting your body go without quality fuel will stunt your progress if not completely stop it. There really is no point hammering away in the gym to not provide your body with the right nutrients to grow. Some nutritionists say the correct diet is 50% of training, others rate it as high as 90%! Yes 90% of what you look like is down to diet, and 10% training. I'd personally say it's more of a 40% training, 60% diet. It's too easy to eat junk after training and use the training to justify it. If we want to build a quality physique, we must be prepared to go all the way.

How much protein do you need?
The RDA is 0.8 grams per kilogram of lean bodyweight (U.S. Food and Nutrition Board, 1980) for sedentary adults (1 kilogram=2.2 pounds)
However you should be aiming for 1.5- 2.4 grams of protein per kilogram of bodyweight. More towards the 2.4 grams will have a maximal effect on building muscle.

Many of the bodybuilders, trainers, and nutritionists agree on these rough figures. Ultimately you will need to find out how your body responds to more protein.

Let's move on to tactics for preparation.

The Big Shop
Firstly you can do a big shop on a Sunday and buy enough food to last until the following Sunday. How much exactly will depend on your nutritional needs. But I'd look at the meals and buy a fair amount. Once you've done a

few shops you'll know exactly what you need. Then you can prepare meals on the Sunday for the next few days so you're not caught short.

3 Day Shop
Another way is to buy enough food to last from Sunday until Wednesday and prepare meals for all those days on the Sunday. Then on the Wednesday I would plan and buy ingredients for Thursday through to Sunday. You will then never find yourself short of key foods to help keep your macro-nutrients at optimal level. Once you've done this a few times it will become second nature and you'll always have the right food to hand.

Something I do now is buy all my fruit and vegetables from the local market. Firstly the prices are much cheaper, but the quality is superb. It's all fresh and delicious. Plus if you eat eggs you can buy those too from a farmer.

So that's the end of my book! I just wanted to thank you for checking out my book and i hope you enjoy the recipes here. Please give my book a review, it really helps me and allows me to continue to write useful content for us Veggies.

These recipes are guides for you to experiment with. More importantly i hope they help you with your muscle building gains and while keeping you living a healthy vegetarian lifestyle.

-Greg

Printed in Great Britain
by Amazon